in the Kitchen

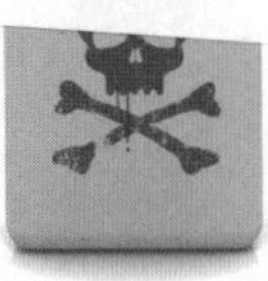

By Joe Crews

CHAPTER 1
Health—A Prime Interest

Some years ago a survey was taken in a certain American city, and every inhabitant responded to 156 questions included in the survey. It was discovered that the prime interest of adults was that of health—not politics, history, or even the weather—but health, their health and the health of their families. What a paradoxical age is this one in which we live! A time when we have more doctors, hospitals, medicines; more medical knowledge of the care, treatment, and cure of disease; more pills, capsules, vitamins, etc.; yet seldom has there been a time when more sickness and general ill health has plagued the human family.

Millions are suffering the side effects of wrong living habits and harmful eating and drinking. We live in a world shattered by pain. The cries of the sick and diseased are the trademarks of modem society. In spite of incredible programs in medical research, the problems of health and longevity are still the most serious our society faces.

The Bible gives a simple, concise answer to the question of premature disability and death.

Millions would still be alive today had they but heeded the warning of God in Exodus 15:26: "If thou wilt diligently hearken to the voice of the Lord thy God, and wilt do that which is right in his sight, and wilt give ear to his commandments, and keep all his statutes, I will put none of these diseases upon thee, which I have brought upon the Egyptians: for I am the Lord that healeth thee."

These words make it abundantly clear that anyone can actually postpone his own funeral. By obeying the laws of God concerning health and diet, disease may be mitigated or avoided altogether. It is apparent from this verse in the Bible that it is not the will of God for great, epidemic scourges to sweep millions into their graves. He wants us to prosper and be in health—body, mind and soul.

Why then do we see so much suffering and disease in the world today? The answer is that the majority are violating the laws of their being. Just as surely as the laws of nature operate, so there are laws of our body that are also predictable and certain. "Whatsoever a man soweth, that shall he also reap" (Galatians 6:7). If a person falls from the roof, the law of gravity immediately takes over. Regardless of age, sex, or financial status, that falling body will hurtle downward to be injured or killed. In the same way, if we violate the laws of our body, we may expect the inevitable consequences of sickness or death.

Effect is always preceded by a cause. To those who have seriously studied the counsels of God and the current world health trends, there is no deep mystery. Experts are puzzled that cancer has continued its spiraling increase. While many diseases have been greatly reduced, and some eliminated altogether, cancer has mushroomed. Even with unprecedented funding and research there have been few significant breakthroughs in curbing the growth of this deadly malignancy.

We can easily understand the steady increase of lung cancer in the light of America's smoking practices. This trend will doubtless continue until more people muster the simple, moral courage to say "no" to imbibing a deadly poison. But few people understand that fully one-third of all cancers of the human body occur within the stomach. And one-half of all cancers are found in the organs of digestion, including the liver, pancreas, small intestine and colon.

The reason for this cancer concentration must be obvious to all of us. Except for the lungs, which are bombarded with hot tobacco tars, the stomach is the most abused organ of the body. Dr. James Ewing, one of the founders of the American Cancer Society, made this statement in a tract entitled The Prevention of Cancer: "The perpetual abuse of a normal stomach frequently gives rise to cancer, and an abnormally weak stomach may suffer the same fate from less abuse. In both instances abuse and overfunction must be regarded as the exciting cause. The stomach is not lined with copper but by a single row of rather delicate epithelial cells. The sole safe conclusion to be drawn from these data is that all forms of abuse of the stomach must be avoided if the high mortality from this very common disease is to be reduced."

It is simply hair-raising and blood-curdling to see what goes into the stomachs of American men, women and children. The great test seems to be whether it tastes good, or else whether it gives a pleasant aftereffect. No wonder 50 percent of the population is suffering from obesity and that more than three million dollars are spent each year on diet formulas and exercise gadgets.

The amazing fact is that the average American consumes 1,488 pounds of food every year. This is undoubtedly a large factor in the one and a half million patients who fill American hospitals every day of the year. Have you ever noticed that three-fifths of the word DEATH is EAT?

Paul Bragg, in his famous cookbook, stated: "The average person is poisoning himself day by day with the food he eats. Most people eat with their eyes. If the food looks good, they do not question whether it is healthful or death-dealing. Few people know the right kind of food to put into their bodies to keep them well and strong or take the time to select this food if they do know. From birth to old age the average individual never experiences the taste of real natural food. Our tiny sensitive taste buds have been for generations so polluted by unnatural, artificially seasoned and stimulating foods that most of us are unable to appreciate the fine, delicate flavor of the natural foods. Foods must be fixed, hashed, mashed, smashed, boiled, broiled, stewed, baked, pickled, preserved, flavored, salted, creamed, dried, roasted, fried, greased, peppered, vinegar-laden, smoked, toasted, crushed, rolled, mealed, oiled, fermented, beaten, sweetened, spiced, soured, peeled, shredded, steamed, braised, colored and otherwise seasoned in order to offer an appeal to the civilized man." Then, he adds, "Civilized man is not satisfied with the food the Maker has supplied him and must do something with it before he feels it is fit for him to eat."

Small wonder, then, that 25 tons of aspirin are swallowed every day in the United States. According to the National Observer, this is 2¼ tablets for every man, woman and child in the nation; and that is every day of the week. If you didn't get your 2¼ tablets today, somebody else got a double supply, you can be sure of that!

One of the strangest paradoxes of American life is found in this area of health. Though people fear sickness above every other enemy, yet they do almost nothing about taking care of their health until after the disease has already struck. In a year's time, out of every medical dollar spent by the American people, 95 cents was spent to get well and five cents were spent on preventive medicine. Now this doesn't make much sense. But in this field most people don't seem to excel in reason or good sense anyway.

It reminds me of a group of tourists in Spain who had gone there to visit one of the historic sites. Up on the side of a cliff, there was an ancient monastery that they wanted to visit. The only way to get up there was in a basket pulled up over a pulley by some of the monks. After they had toured the monastery, they were being lowered back down the side of the cliff. As they were getting into the basket to be lowered back down, they noticed that the rope was rather frayed. So they asked the monk in charge, "How often do you change the rope?" And the monk said, "Well, we change it every time it breaks, of course." That wasn't much comfort to those who were being lowered down in the basket.

More and more, the medical researchers are finding out that our diet has very much to do with our state of health. The body machine is actually made up of the fuel we feed into it. The quality of nerve, bone, blood and cell is dependent upon good nutrition and proper diet. The old adage is almost literally true: Millions are digging their graves with their teeth.

CHAPTER 2
Our Bodies Not Our Own

Right at this point someone may be wondering what all this has to do with religion. Why would God be concerned about my eating habits? Isn't it a man's personal business as to how he cares for his body? These are relevant questions and cannot be ignored.

Fortunately, the Creator of our bodies did not leave us without answers to these questions. "Whether therefore ye eat, or drink, or whatsoever ye do, do all to the glory of God" (1 Corinthians 10:31). Isn't that amazing? God is concerned about such small matters as what and how and when we feed our body system. The Bible reveals that God did not fabricate the delicate human machine and then leave it to operate alone. He has never released His ownership of the creative process or of the product itself.

The apostle Paul wrote: "What? know ye not that your body is the temple of the Holy Ghost which is in you, which ye have of God, and ye are not your own? For ye are bought with a price: therefore glorify God in your body, and in your spirit, which are God's" (1 Corinthians 6:19, 20). These words reveal that the proper care of our body is not only a spiritual obligation but a moral requirement. Even though we have control of our bodies, they do not really belong to us. We are only stewards of someone else's property.

No man has a right to say, "I'll do as I please with my own body, and it is my business alone." We can rob God by violating the divine purpose of the body temple be the dwelling place of the Holy Spirit.

Paul refers to both the church and the individual member when he says: "Know ye not that ye are the temple of God, and that the Spirit of God dwelleth in you? If any man defile the temple of God, him shall God destroy; for the temple of God is holy, which temple ye are" (1 Corinthians 3:16, 17). This forever settles that a person can be lost for defiling the property of God.

But how much does the average individual know about his own body and how to take care of it? Doesn't it seem strange to you that the average parent knows more about the physical needs of the chickens in the pen, or a dog in the house, than he does about the needs of his own children? The average man knows more about the needs of his automobile than he does about the physical needs of his own family! Why is there such an incredible amount of ignorance concerning the way to take care of this sacred body temple? The Bible assures us that the human body is to be cared for, preserved and maintained according to the rules laid down in the Bible. The trouble is that most Americans simply follow their appetite in matters of eating and drinking.

What are the guidelines laid down in the Bible about caring for and feeding the body? God asks the question, "Wherefore do ye spend money for that which is not bread? and your labor for that which satisfieth not? … eat ye that which is good" (Isaiah 55:2). And how can we tell what is good? Surely not by the taste or the advertising or by colorful labels. Most Americans, following the law of appetite, hastily fill their grocery baskets with the products that have been most loudly touted by the TV hawkers. With no regard to content, they collect everything that appeals to the taste and sight. As little baby birds open their mouths to whatever mama will put in, so the gullible consumers blindly accept the choices of the media marketers.

CHAPTER 3
Body Maker's Manual

There is only one way to know what is good for this very complex body system, and that is to consult the One who made it. Only the manufacturer has the best operating manual for its products. Automobile makers always provide such instructions for keeping their vehicles in top running condition.

When God made the body, He also gave specific operating instructions, including fuel and maintenance. Notice this counsel in Genesis 1:29, "Behold, I have given you every herb bearing seed, which is upon the face of all the earth, and every tree, in the which is the fruit of a tree yielding seed; to you it shall be for meat." No one has been able to improve on it. Nuts, fruits, grains and vegetables are still recognized by the best nutritionists as the finest possible diet.

No one need be reluctant to espouse the ideal vegetarian diet commanded by a perfect God for the perfect bodies He created in the beginning. Today, under the increasing curse of sin, those bodies have degenerated in both size and stamina, but no argument or scientific data has been able to challenge the wisdom of God's original arrangement.

But notice how the American people have departed from the simplicity of that original recipe. Today the average eater's plate is loaded with heavy meat protein, carbohydrates and pastries. In the beginning, God did not even allow for the use of meat. Apparently flesh was permitted in man's diet for the first time only after the flood waters had annihilated all vegetable matter—but only certain meats. God gave this instruction to Noah: "Of every clean beast thou shalt take to thee by sevens, the male and his female: and of the beasts that are not clean by two, the male and his female" (Genesis 7:2).

Don't miss the significant fact that the law of clean and unclean animals extends all the way back to the beginning of human history. Many have assumed that only the Jewish people were forbidden to eat the unclean animals. Not so. There were no Jews in Noah's day, yet the distinction is clearly made. Why were extra clean animals taken into the ark?

Because all vegetation would be wiped out in the flood, and for the first time, God would allow man to eat meat.

But only the clean meat! If Noah and his family had eaten any of the unclean animals, that species would have ceased to exist because only a male and female had been preserved to perpetuate the species. There were seven pairs of the clean animals in the ark. Only they could be spared for food without endangering the continuity of their kind.

Since it is evident that even some Genesis-kind animals were unclean, how do we determine where the line is drawn between the clean and unclean? God has not left us to wonder about this important issue.

In Leviticus 11:3–11 the requirements are clearly laid out: "Whatsoever parteth the hoof, and is clovenfooted, and cheweth the cud, among the beasts, that shall ye eat. Nevertheless these shall ye not eat of them that chew the cud, or of them that divide the hoof: as the camel, because he cheweth the cud, but divideth not the hoof; he is unclean unto you. And the coney, because he cheweth the cud, but divideth not the hoof; he is unclean unto you. And the hare, because he cheweth the cud, but divideth not the hoof; he is unclean unto you. And the swine, though he divide the hoof, and be clovenfooted, yet he cheweth not the cud; he is unclean to you. … These shall ye eat of all that are in the waters: whatsoever hath fins and scales in the waters, in the seas, and in the rivers, them shall ye eat. And all that have not fins and scales in the seas, and in the rivers, of all that move in the waters, and of any living thing which is in the waters, they shall be an abomination unto you … ye shall not eat of their flesh."

CHAPTER 4
Pork Unclean

How fortunate we are that the One who made us also prescribed the kind of food that should and should not be eaten. We may not be able to explain why some are unclean and others clean, but we can trust the Creator to know the difference, and in His great love for us He has revealed it for our good. All animals that do not have a split hoof and chew the cud are not to be eaten.

Is it any surprise to us that Satan has created an appetite for the very foods God forbade? And should it be any surprise that epidemic disease has followed the violation of God's dietary principles? The forbidden swine is a perfect example of how presumptuous appetite has overruled God's sensible restrictions. Unlike some of the other unclean categories, we can show abundant scientific evidence why pork is totally unfit for food.

Pork contains a microscopic worm called trichina, and if it gets into the system, the disease trichinosis results. Governments warn that there is no inspection for the parasite, and a *Readers' Digest* article stresses that there is no cure for the disease.

Under the title "Must Our Pork Remain Unsafe?" these statements are made about trichinosis: "A single serving of defective pork, even a single mouthful, can kill or cripple or condemn the victim to a lifetime of aches and pains. For this unique disease, trichinosis, there is no cure. With no drugs to stop them the worms may spread through the entire muscular tissues of the human system.

"One of two things then happens, depending on the intensity of the infection. Either death ensues or a successful effort is made by nature to throw an enclosure, or cyst, around each of the teeming parasites, which then become dormant, although they remain alive for years. Don't blame your doctor. All that the best doctor can do as yet is to conserve the patient's strength and try to relieve the painful, local symptoms as they appear" (*Reader's Digest*, March 1950). What these symptoms are, the layman had much better not worry about. Trichinosis can simulate to some degree almost any other malady. That pain in your arm or leg may be arthritis or rheumatism or it may be trichinosis. That pain in your back may mean a gall bladder involvement, but it may mean trichinosis.

Dr. Samuel C. Gould, a Washington health official, who has made an extensive study of trichinosis, states that the average American consumer eats at least 200 infested pork meals during his lifetime. Just because the meat may be stamped "U.S. Government Inspected and Passed" does not mean it has been tested for trichina infestation. Every bit of the pork would have to go under a microscope to make that determination.

The Public Health Service advises consumers to cook the pork thoroughly in order to kill the trichina worms. Someone has observed that eating dead worms is not very highly appealing to the palate either. The act is that God calls it unclean and an abomination. Why is it so hard for Christians to accept the judgment of God over the perverted craving of appetite?

Some have asked why God created the pig if it should not be eaten. The answer to that is self-evident. The pigs, along with buzzards, snakes and hyenas, are great scavengers of the earth's filth and refuse. All creatures serve a purpose, but all are not suitable for assimilation into the human system as food. We might not be able to figure that out in our own wisdom, but the counsels of God have revealed it beyond all doubt or question.

Arguments have been advanced that there is better sanitation since God made those Old Testament laws, and the pig is now quite fit to be eaten. One is hard put to believe that land or sea animals have become less polluted by the passing of time. Today there are chemical poisons infecting land, sea, and atmosphere to such an alarming degree that constant government directives are being issued. Environmentalists keep us posted hour by hour on the massive accumulation of deadly pesticides, insecticides, and other contaminants in every order of nature.

And if reason doesn't convince us that the unclean animals are still unclean, we have the revelation of God's Word on the matter. Isaiah writes: "For, behold, the Lord will come with fire, and with his chariots like a whirlwind, to render his anger with fury, and his rebuke with flames of fire. For by fire and by his sword will the Lord plead with all flesh: and the slain of the Lord shall be many. They that sanctify themselves, and purify themselves in the gardens behind one tree in the midst, eating swine's flesh, and the abomination, and the mouse, shall be consumed together, saith the Lord" (Isaiah 66:15–17).

This text is talking about the second coming of Jesus and proves that the nature of those animals will not experience any change that will make them fit to eat—not even down to the very last day of this earth when Jesus comes. The swine is placed in the same category as the abomination and mouse, and God plainly declares that the eaters thereof "shall be consumed together." None can say that the warning has not been given in language that everyone can understand.

CHAPTER 5
Seafood Not Fit to Eat

It should be noted that only the marine animals that have fins and scales are counted as "clean" in Leviticus 11. All others are an abomination to God. This eliminates oysters, shrimp, crabs, clams, eels, catfish, lobsters and crayfish. Again, the scavengers have been forbidden as articles of diet.

Are there sound, scientific reasons for accepting God's appraisal of these shellfish and other seafood? It is quite common knowledge that these creatures feed largely on the raw sewage and pollutants in the water.

Prevention magazine of September 1972, carried an interesting article entitled "Shellfish Are Dirty and Dangerous." The author appeared reluctant to take a stand, but he was committed to telling the truth on this sensitive subject. He wrote: "They're succulent; they're delicious; they're even nutritious. But, because of the nature of the mollusk and the sewage-like pollution of its habitat, we must in good conscience advise you to avoid shellfish, no matter how they tempt you, and even though those around you seem to be swallowing them with delight. The day of reckoning cometh.

"Why are shellfish so dangerous? Because they are many times more polluted than the filthy waters they inhabit.

"Unfortunately they choose to live and love and multiply in estuaries along coastal regions. These estuaries are particularly subject to discharge of sewage, sewage effluent, and other water-borne pollution from municipal discharges, from suburban home drainage and agricultural runoff.

"The polluted aspect of their habitat is one danger. The fact that they are filter feeders compounds the danger.

"Oysters, for instance, because of their way of obtaining and absorbing food, have been found to concentrate polio virus up to 20 to 60 times the level of the surrounding seawater.

"No other animal food offered on the menu of your favorite eating place would be served to you along with its feces. Yet this is the case with seafood. It is served whole; complete with its intestinal tract."

Can you imagine anyone finding such fare to be a culinary delicacy? Over and over again outbreaks of hepatitis have been traced to the eating of seafood. After feeding on raw sewage, the creature is harvested and sold. The disease is simply cycled from man to mollusk and then back to man.

Again we must confess the loving concern of an all-knowing God for the health and happiness of His creation. And those who deliberately flaunt the divine laws will finally suffer the tragic consequence that disobedience always produces.

CHAPTER 6
Alcohol—A Curse

Now let us consider how to glorify God in what we drink or inhale into the body. The Bible says, "Whether therefore ye eat, or drink,... do all to the glory of God" (1 Corinthians 10:31). Among all the popular poisons which are imbibed by modern man, one that is particularly pernicious and destructive is alcohol. Glorified as a symbol of gracious living, it has, in fact, been the most malignant social disease known to civilization. No wonder the Bible declares that no drunkard will be in heaven.

In these days of compromise, most of the great religious bodies have changed their attitude toward social drinking. From total abstinence they now take a stance of moderation. In essence this is exactly the same position the brewers take—no drunkenness. But is that a safe posture to take toward alcoholic beverages? Statistics reveal that one out of every ten that start drinking become either alcoholics or problem drinkers.

The claim is made by many Christians that the Bible endorses moderate drinking of alcohol. This is based largely on the use of the term "wine" in the Scriptures. But the recommended wine of the Bible is not alcoholic. The word wine is used for either fermented or unfermented drink. God declared, "As the new wine is found in the cluster, and one saith, Destroy it not; for a blessing is in it: so will I do for my servants' sakes, that I may not destroy them" (Isaiah 65:8).

This wine in the cluster has to be the fresh juice of the vine. This is the only kind God ever declared to have a blessing in it. There is no blessing in the intoxicating, befuddling bottle of fermented poison. Inspiration declares, "Wine is a mocker, strong drink is raging: and whosoever is deceived thereby is not wise"

(Proverbs 20:1). "Look not thou upon the wine when it is red, when it giveth his color in the cup, when it moveth itself aright. At the last it biteth like a serpent, and stingeth like an adder" (Proverbs 23:31, 32).

Did Jesus go contrary to the Old Testament and turn the water into alcoholic wine? It is unthinkable that He should do so. He obeyed the Word of God. The wine He created was the unfermented kind. We now know the actual physiological effect of alcohol on the body. Research has proven that intoxication is caused by a process that deprives the brain of oxygen. This deprivation destroys brain cells, affecting, ultimately, the reasoning powers of conscious thought. Would Jesus, the Creator of the body, condone something that would weaken moral inhibitions, reduce the power of effective decision, and finally destroy the sacred body temple of the Holy Spirit? Never. And what can we say about the use of tobacco?

CHAPTER 7
Nicotine–Most Deadly Poison

Books could be written about the massive research into the noxious effect of nicotine on the body. Since the Surgeon General's first release on the subject, every new study has documented more supporting information. Nicotine is possibly the most deadly poison known to man. Millions have died as a result of its malignant influence. By constricting the arteries of the body, nicotine forces the heart to overexert. Lungs have become riddled with carcinoma. Fetuses have been fatally affected. Hardly an organ of the body escapes the insidious effect of the fatal nicotine poison.

Is it a sin to use tobacco? There is no sense in denying a patent truth. Anything that defiles the holy body sanctuary is a sin. God says He will destroy those who do it. We dare not call it less than it is. It is a sin, and no Christian should presumptuously shorten his life by introducing it into his body.

Few church members would consider taking even small, microscopic doses of arsenic or strychnine into their body, yet they take something just as lethal. Slowly the cigarette tars coat the delicate membranes of the lungs until death results. It is exactly the same when men and women deliberately inhale the toxic fumes of tobacco until the cumulative effect causes death. It is suicide on the installment plan. It is morally wrong to take God's property, violate our stewardship, and rob Him of His possessions.

And what can we say about the waste of money on tobacco? Most smokers spend $50 or more every month for their indulgence. By retirement time this would amount to $25,000. Enough to guarantee a late-life nest egg, even if Social Security fails. Yet many of those who waste that money on tobacco come to the end of life penniless and dependent on welfare or relatives. What an unspeakable tragedy! No wonder God said, "My people are destroyed for lack of knowledge" (Hosea 4:6). How much better it would be to simply place the $25,000 in a neat pile and strike a match to it. At least it would not be serving as a destroyer of life.

We can surely see by now what a serious matter it is to desecrate the physical body and mind created for a specific, spiritual purpose. This principle of being accountable to God for the way we take care of our bodies is rooted deeply in the Bible, but millions are becoming health conscious today just to avoid the painful effects of neglecting their bodies. And it is so true that reason and good judgment alone should provide enough motivation for a balanced diet and exercise program.

But sometimes logic, and even scientific evidence, has a tremendous conflict with appetite, social custom and addiction. Caffeine is a dramatic example. There is a growing catalog of research that points to caffeine as a pernicious enemy of good health. It is a powerful, habit-forming drug that has fastened millions in a vise of addiction. Many find it just as hard to give up caffeinated drinks as to stop smoking or drinking. It has been indicted for its adverse effect upon heart, stomach, nerves and even the fetuses of expectant mothers.

CHAPTER 8
Coffee Drunkards

Merck Index of Drugs lists quite a variety of caffeine symptoms and indicates that seven grains of the drug is a medical dose. Most cola drinks, tea, and coffee contain from one and a half to three grains. Many people take far more than a medical dose at every meal. The effect is to stimulate the cells of the body to operate on a higher level of activity than God ever intended. One physician described it this way: "We in America have become a nation of tea and coffee drunkards."

Incredible as it seems, this country consumes 275 billion pounds of coffee every year. That averages 17 pounds for every man, woman and child. Doctors warn heart patients and those with stomach ulcers to leave off caffeine, along with smoking. Another coffee factor has recently been established as cancer-causing. This is, by far, the most serious charge that has grown out of the coffee research. Although the carcinogen has not been identified as caffeine, it is definitely associated with coffee drinking.

Tea, in addition to its content of caffeine, has another harmful constituent, tannic acid. This powerful chemical is used for dyeing leather. The detrimental effect of sugar concentration in the caffeinated drinks provides still another reason for eliminating it from the diet. The murderous effect of refined sugar threatens the well-being of every habitual user of soft drinks.

It is not uncommon to see secretaries or bosses sitting at their desks with a cigarette in one hand, a cup of coffee nearby, and a Coca-Cola on the credenza. Who hasn't heard their common rationale: "If I don't get my coffee (or coke) I get a headache"? They are telling the truth. The caffeine does take away the headache, but so would a tenth of a grain of morphine. The temporary, sedative effect is to deaden the pain, but the daily dosing of delicate nerve-endings wears off, leaving them more jangled, and demanding more and more sedation.

The most pathetic proof of this drug-slavery is to be found in expectant mothers. With all the accumulation of medical data proving the damaging effect of alcohol, tobacco and caffeine on the fetuses, pregnant women still pour the poison into the bodies of their unborn babies. It might be possible to understand a woman willing to risk her own life and health by a perverse indulgence in chemical poisons, but how could she so deliberately endanger the life of her child? The answer to that question reveals the depth of the drug problem in American society.

CHAPTER 9
The Big Question

The big question, of course, is how to quit. After the will has been weakened by years of indulgence, how does one find the power to resist the powerful craving for these narcotic-type drugs? Most will only find deliverance from outside themselves. First, there must be a decision to stop—a willingness to give up the physical pleasure associated with the habit. All available effort should be mustered for the conflict. Then pray. Claim the mighty promises of the Bible for total victory.

Don't try to taper off on the use of something that is morally and physically wrong to indulge. It just doesn't work. It is much like cutting off the dog's tail a little at a time to make it easier on the dog! It is actually more painful that way. A habit is a habit. If you cut off the "h" you still have "abit" left. Take off the "a" and "bit" remains. Remove the "b" and "it" is still with you. Even after taking away the "i" you are left with "t." And if your problem is tea-drinking, you still don't have the full victory.

Someone may object that we are trying to take away too much. After all, you can overdo anything. Too many potatoes or beans can also be very harmful to some people. Indeed they can, and a true definition of temperance should read like this: A total abstinence from things that are harmful, and a moderate, judicious use of the things that are good. Doesn't that make a lot of sense? It also contains a lot of good, sound religion.

Impressive evidence that a person can postpone his own funeral was presented by Paul Harvey in his news column. Under the title Eat Right, Live Longer, Harvey described the results of a western survey on longevity. The study focused on the death certificates of California Seventh-day Adventists in comparison to non-SDAs. Comparing the records of the Adventist (who teach against drinking, smoking, or using caffeine) with others, the survey revealed that Seventh-day Adventists have a life expectancy almost six years greater than other Californians.

Seventy percent fewer Adventists die from all types of cancer, 68 percent fewer from respiratory disease, 88 percent fewer from TB and 85 percent fewer from pulmonary emphysema. Adventists have 46 percent less strokes, 60 percent less heart disease. Perhaps as a by-product of abstinence from alcohol, they have only about one-third as many accidents.

Again we are faced with the reassuring truth that all of us can add years to our lives by simply obeying the practical, ageless principles laid down by our Creator in the Bible. Rather than feeling cheated or short-changed, we ought to rejoice that God loves us enough to share with us His secrets of long life and happiness. The apostle John wrote, "Beloved, now are we the sons of God, and it doth not yet appear what we shall be: but we know that, when he shall appear, we shall be like him, for we shall see him as he is. And every man that hath this hope in him purifieth himself, even as he is pure" (1 John 3:2, 3).

Do you have the faith and courage to accept the inspired prescription that can lengthen your life and tranquility? Seize it right now as the course that can prepare you well for both time and eternity.